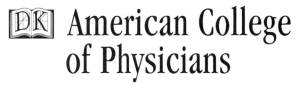

American College of Physicians

HOME MEDICAL GUIDE *to*

URINARY INCONTINENCE IN WOMEN

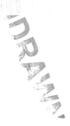

D0931934

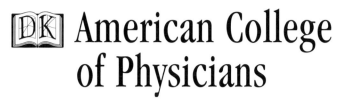

American College
of Physicians

HOME MEDICAL GUIDE *to*

URINARY
INCONTINENCE
IN WOMEN

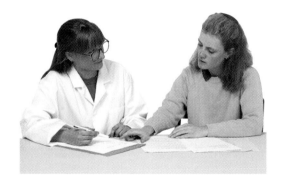

MEDICAL EDITOR
DAVID R. GOLDMANN, MD
ASSOCIATE MEDICAL EDITOR
DAVID A. HOROWITZ, MD

A DORLING KINDERSLEY BOOK

IMPORTANT

The American College of
Physicians (ACP) Home Medical
Guides provide general
information on a wide range of
health and medical topics. These
books are not substitutes for
medical diagnosis, and you should
always consult your doctor on
personal health matters before
undertaking any program of
therapy or treatment. Various
medical organizations have
different guidelines for diagnosis
and treatment of the same
conditions; the American College
of Physicians–American Society of
Internal Medicine (ACP–ASIM)
has tried to present a reasonable
consensus of these opinions.

Material in this book was
reviewed by the ACP–ASIM for
general medical accuracy and
applicability in the United States;
however, the information provided
herein does not necessarily reflect
the specific recommendations
or opinions of the ACP–ASIM.
The naming of any organization,
product, or alternative therapy in
these books is not an ACP–ASIM
endorsement, and the omission of
any such name does not indicate
ACP–ASIM disapproval.

DORLING KINDERSLEY
LONDON, NEW YORK, AUCKLAND, DELHI,
JOHANNESBURG, MUNICH, PARIS, AND SYDNEY

www.dk.com

Senior Editors Jill Hamilton, Nicki Lampon
Senior Designer Jan English
DTP Design Jason Little
Editor Ashley Ren
Medical Consultant Mary Ann Forceia, MD

Senior Managing Editor Martyn Page
Senior Managing Art Editor Bryn Walls

Published in the United States in 2000 by
Dorling Kindersley Publishing, Inc.,
95 Madison Avenue, New York, New York 10016

2 4 6 8 10 9 7 5 3 1

Library of Congress Catalog Card Number 99-76855
ISBN 0-7894-4171-3

Reproduced by Colourscan, Singapore
Printed and bound in the United States by Quebecor World, Taunton, Massachusetts

Contents

What is incontinence?

Urinary incontinence is defined as involuntary loss of urine and often causes social or hygienic problems. It is a common condition that is embarrassing and distressing and may severely affect your quality of life.

Incontinence may be quite mild – the occasional leaking of small amounts amounts of urine that does not cause embarrassment and that would therefore not be considered a problem – or it can be very severe. People with a severe problem may have to wear pads constantly to stay dry, avoid normal activities such as sports, and worry about people noticing the smell of urine.

The causes of incontinence are varied, and some are easily corrected, just as constipation can be easily cured by a better diet or a urinary infection can be treated with antibiotics. Others may require surgery or long-term medication.

This book was written to help you learn about incontinence and how it can be treated. It is not designed to

WOMEN WITH CHILDREN
Incontinence is far more commonly found in women, particularly those who have given birth, although it can also affect men and children.

replace a consultation with your doctor, but we hope that it will help you understand the problem better. It also discusses other urinary disorders, such as recurrent cystitis and bladder pain, because not all women with bladder problems experience leakage.

WHO IS AFFECTED?

Urinary incontinence is most commonly found in women who have had children, but it can also affect children, men, and women who have never had children. Recent studies suggest that up to 30 percent of all women and over 60 percent of patients in nursing homes may be affected. However, this is probably an underestimate, since many women may be too embarrassed to admit that they have a problem.

WHAT ARE THE SYMPTOMS?

In addition to leakage, there is a range of other symptoms of urinary incontinence and bladder problems. You may have to urinate more often than usual, which is known as frequency, and it may be painful or difficult to do so, which is called dysuria. You may have a sudden and uncontrollable need to urinate. This is called urgency and can lead to leakage if you are unable to reach a toilet in time. All three are common symptoms of cystitis, an inflammation of the bladder. You may have to get up in the night to urinate, which is known as nocturia, or you may have difficulties emptying the bladder, known as voiding problems. You may have the sensation of wanting to urinate but be unable to do so at will, or you may suffer from hesitancy, which is a delay before urination begins.

WHERE TO GO FOR HELP

Currently, the average period of time before a woman seeks medical help for incontinence is five years. She may be embarrassed by the problem or feel that it is to be expected after having children, and she may think that nothing can be done. Or she may learn various strategies to "manage" the problem, for example, by emptying her bladder frequently to prevent accumulation of enough urine to leak.

You should be reassured that there is a great deal of help available from your doctor and from specialist incontinence clinics. There are many treatment options, and they range from simple changes in lifestyle to surgery. Some improvement in symptoms is possible for nearly everyone with incontinence. Help can also be given in managing the symptoms more effectively.

Case History 1: STRESS INCONTINENCE

Sarah Hunt is a 36-year-old woman who has had difficulties with urine leaking when she coughed. Her problems started after the birth of her second child when she was 30. At first, she noticed slight leakage when doing aerobics, causing her to stop doing the step exercises. Over the next three years, the problem worsened, and she stopped going to the gym entirely. She eventually went to her doctor for help after the problem became so bad that she leaked in public when she picked up her daughter. When she saw

MEDICAL HELP
Sarah sought medical advice for her stress incontinence problems after she began to leak in public.

her doctor, she was wearing sanitary napkins whenever she went out, and her friends had a standing joke about her always going to the bathroom before leaving home.

Sarah was referred to her local hospital, where she underwent urodynamics tests that showed stress incontinence. At this time, Sarah was unsure whether she wanted more children and was therefore referred to an advanced practice nurse, who taught her Kegel exercises. After four months of these exercises, she was able to control her problem. When she goes to the gym now, she wears a large vaginal tampon that prevents leakage during aerobics classes.

MAKING LIFE EASIER
Dorothy's urge incontinence problems were improved by bladder drill therapy and the use of the drug oxybutynin.

Case History 2: **URGE INCONTINENCE**

Dorothy Evans is a 65-year-old woman who went to see her doctor because she was often going to the bathroom to urinate. When she was shopping, she felt that if she did not urinate frequently she would leak and occasionally she did. Her doctor ordered a supply of incontinence pads and recommended that she be assessed at her local hospital. The urodynamics tests showed detrusor instability.

Dorothy started taking oxybutynin and began bladder drill behavioral therapy (see pp.43–45). She can now manage to go shopping without using the bathroom, and she no longer needs to carry changes of underwear in case she leaks.

KEY POINTS

- Incontinence is a common problem.
- It leads to a range of symptoms.
- Women are often reluctant to seek help.
- There is a great deal of help available.

How the bladder works

It is important to understand how the bladder works because there are many different types of incontinence that may have different causes and may therefore respond to different forms of treatment.

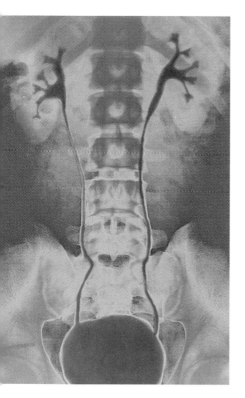

URINARY SYSTEM
This X-ray shows the kidneys (at the top), the bladder (at the bottom), and the ureters (ducts connecting the kidneys to the bladder).

BLADDER ANATOMY

The bladder consists of a flexible sac of muscle (the detrusor muscle). Urine is produced in the kidneys and passes into the bladder through the ureters. The urine is then stored in the bladder until it is released during urination. During storage, the urine is retained in the bladder by a ring of muscles at the bottom of the bladder called the urethral sphincter, which squeezes shut. The bladder neck, the area where the bladder and urethra meet, is partly supported in its position by the pelvic floor muscles. These muscles form a sling in the pelvis that helps support the bladder, vagina, and rectum.

The pelvic floor helps hold the urethra in position on the underside of the pelvic bone. When you cough

Location of the Bladder in Women

The bladder is a muscle-lined sac situated in the lower abdomen. Its function is to store urine (liquid filtered from the bloodstream by the kidneys and then transferred to the bladder by the ureters) until the time of urination.

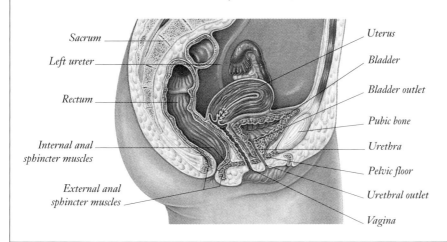

Sacrum
Left ureter
Rectum
Internal anal sphincter muscles
External anal sphincter muscles

Uterus
Bladder
Bladder outlet
Pubic bone
Urethra
Pelvic floor
Urethral outlet
Vagina

or sneeze, the increased pressure in the abdomen is transmitted both to the urethra and the bladder. Since the pressure on the urethra keeps it closed in the normal situation, the bladder does not usually leak when you cough or sneeze. This principle is known as the pressure transmission theory, and it forms the basis of our understanding of continence. The pressure transmission theory is also the principle on which most surgical operations for incontinence are based.

Bladder function is highly complex. It requires coordination from several parts of the brain and involves both involuntary and voluntary activity. This can be illustrated by looking in more detail at the urethral sphincter. It is made up of two parts, each with its own

13

function. The inner sphincter is made up of involuntary muscle that the brain operates without conscious thought. This muscle maintains a constant steady pressure, squeezing the urethra closed. It is helped by the lining of the urethra, which is folded inward many times so that it forms a watertight seal when it is compressed. The outer sphincter is made up of muscle that is under more voluntary control, and it is this, along with the pelvic floor, that can be consciously squeezed when trying to prevent leakage. It is capable of very strong contractions but for only a short period of time. The muscle can be fatigued, and this is why a sneezing fit may cause leakage after only the third or fourth sneeze.

BLADDER CONTROL

Reflex Action
A baby has no control over his or her bladder. It empties involuntarily about once an hour.

A newborn baby will empty his or her bladder about once an hour under reflex control, which means that the bladder empties automatically when it feels full. This involves only the bladder and the nerves running between the bladder and the spinal cord; at this stage, the brain is not involved. The sensory nerves are stimulated by the filling of the bladder. These nerves go to the spinal cord, where they are connected to the motor nerves, which go back to the bladder and cause it to contract. At the same time, the urethra relaxes, allowing urine to pass out of the bladder. Therefore, the bladder fills and then empties; it is not yet used for storage.

14

As a baby gets older (about the age of two years), its brain develops and starts to intercept the messages from the sensory nerves. The brain can then suppress the impulse to make the bladder muscle contract and can stop the reflexive emptying of the bladder. The capacity of the bladder will then increase, and it develops into a storage organ. In the course of toilet training, we learn what is acceptable behavior and start to use the parts of our brain that are connected with bladder control.

Higher brain functions may also affect bladder function. An example of this effect is the desire of some people to urinate when they hear running water.

TOILET TRAINING
A child gains more control over urination as the nerves in the bladder mature, and the bladder capacity gradually increases.

BLADDER FUNCTION

Bladder function can be thought of as having two distinct phases: filling and storage of urine, and emptying the bladder of urine (voiding).

In filling, the urethra is squeezed shut while the bladder itself is relaxed, expanding as it fills with urine. In voiding, the urethra relaxes just before a contraction of the detrusor muscle in the bladder wall. The urine is then pushed through the urethra to the outside.

How often you urinate depends both on how much urine is produced and how much the bladder will hold. If you drink 8 cups of liquid a day and your bladder normally holds 2 cups, you will empty your bladder approximately four times a day. A bladder that holds only half a cup results in urination 16 times. If you drink twice as much, you will need to empty your bladder twice as frequently.

Normal frequency of urination is up to seven times a day or not more than every two hours. In young women, the bladder normally holds 14 to 20 fluid ounces and is usually emptied when holding 9 to 14 fluid ounces. As people age, bladder capacity tends to decrease, leading to increased frequency of urination, especially at night.

HOW PROBLEMS ARISE

If the bladder neck and urethral sphincters are damaged, which may happen during childbirth, then they will not be as effective at sealing the urine inside the bladder. The bladder neck may also move downward if the structures that support it are weakened, and this will add to the problem. Again, this may result from childbirth, but straining may also be a cause. Straining can result from constipation or a chronic smoker's cough.

The bladder itself may be unstable or overactive, a condition known as detrusor instability. It is not known exactly what causes this, but it may be linked to loss of normal control of the bladder-emptying reflex, nerve damage sustained during childbirth, or previous surgery to treat incontinence.

Anything that interferes with the parts of the brain involved in modifying bladder activity can affect bladder function. For example, a stroke or a spinal injury may interrupt the connection between the higher parts of the brain and the bottom of the spinal cord, resulting in a return to the reflex voiding pattern of a baby, incomplete emptying, or loss of control.

Any kind of mass pressing on the bladder, such as fibroids or a rectum that is full of feces due to constipation, can cause urinary problems that will be discussed in detail later.

KEY POINTS

- Normal bladder control is highly complex.
- Bladder control is learned early in life.
- How often you urinate depends on how much you drink and the capacity of your bladder.
- Continence depends on normal positioning of the bladder neck, normal nerve control of the bladder, and normal coordination and mental state. People who are unconscious or those who have dementia cannot control their bladders.

Why does incontinence affect primarily women?

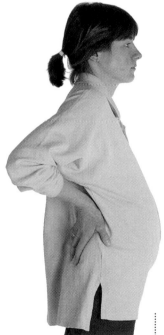

EFFECTS OF PREGNANCY
The physical changes that occur during pregnancy lead to a need to urinate more often.

As we have seen, incontinence is a condition that can affect anyone. However, there are several reasons why women are more prone to it than men are.

PREGNANCY

In pregnancy, the body's systems adapt to provide for the fetus as well as the mother. The bladder and pelvis undergo several changes during this time.

One of the first effects of pregnancy is an increase in the amount of urine produced by the kidneys. This results very early on in an increase in the frequency of urination. Other hormonal effects lead to a general relaxation of the tissues in the pelvis, allowing the pelvis to become more flexible during the pregnancy and birth. The bladder may not empty as well during pregnancy as a result of the pressure effects. These changes may cause a reduction in the natural barriers to bacteria, which can lead to an increased occurrence of urinary tract infections. As the uterus enlarges, increased pressure on the bladder leads to the need to urinate more frequently.

In about one-third of all pregnant women, this increased pressure causes leakage. The leakage usually stops with the birth of the baby and does not lead to incontinence after childbirth.

Pregnancy can also lead to damage of the nerves controlling the muscles in the pelvis. In some women, the damage appears not to heal, and this may be one of the causes of subsequent problems.

CHILDBIRTH

Childbirth can damage the muscles and supporting structures of the pelvis. During a vaginal delivery, there is stretching of the side walls of the vagina and of the muscles of the pelvic floor. These muscles and tissues may not recover completely, and this can cause a loss of support of the uterus and bladder neck that may eventually lead to prolapse of the uterus.

As the baby descends the birth canal, the pudendal nerve, which controls the muscles of the pelvic floor encompassing the edge of the birth canal, may be damaged. This nerve damage may lead to incontinence.

Breast-feeding helps the mother burn off the excess weight put on during pregnancy and passes on important nutrition and antibodies to the baby. It also delays the resumption of menstruation. The delay in return to normal function of the ovaries also means that the amount of circulating estrogen is less than usual. Since the tissues in the pelvis are estrogen-sensitive, this may cause the pelvis to take longer to recover from damage.

Presently, there is no way to predict accurately which women are at risk of developing incontinence after childbirth. Various factors that may influence the effect

BREAST-FEEDING
Estrogen levels may fall during breast-feeding, so that any damage to the estrogen-sensitive tissues in the pelvis caused by giving birth will take longer to heal.

of childbirth on the pelvis include the number of children, the type of delivery, the weight of the babies, the duration of labor, and the length of time the mother pushed. The first vaginal delivery carries the greatest risk, but despite this most women have no long-term symptoms. Assisted deliveries with forceps do carry a higher risk than do normal deliveries. Cesarean section seems to minimize some of these effects, but the benefit is lost after repeated pregnancies.

One thing that does seem to be effective in minimizing the risk of incontinence after childbirth is the performance of Kegel exercises (see Finding out what's wrong, pp.23–28). These exercises must be taught properly

Instrument Deliveries

Special procedures are sometimes necessary during a childbirth. The use of instruments such as forceps to assist in the delivery of a baby increases the risk of the subsequent development of incontinence.

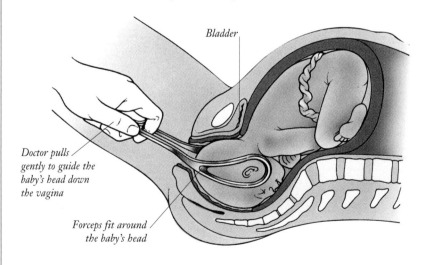

Bladder

Doctor pulls gently to guide the baby's head down the vagina

Forceps fit around the baby's head

and practiced frequently. Most doctors feel that performing Kegel exercises before delivery may help prevent incontinence. They must be continued long afterward to be totally effective.

MENOPAUSE

At menopause, the ovaries cease to function and estrogen levels in the blood fall dramatically. This change can be responsible for the symptoms commonly associated with menopause, such as hot flashes and night sweats. It also has an effect on the pelvic tissues, which are estrogen-sensitive. As estrogen levels drop, the muscles and tissues in the pelvis thin and lose some of their strength. This particularly affects collagen, a supporting protein in the skin. As a result, support of pelvic organs such as the bladder, bowel, and uterus is lost and may eventually cause vaginal prolapse.

Treatment with hormone replacement therapy may help reverse these changes, but it will not cure the problem because, once the collagen has weakened, it will never totally regain its strength.

One other long-term result of low estrogen is atrophic vaginitis, a condition in which the vaginal walls become thin and inflamed, causing itching and soreness. Atrophic vaginitis may be associated with changes in the bacteria within the vagina. The vaginal discomfort may lead to irritation around the urethra and, consequently, to more frequent urination.

BLADDER INFECTION

The pelvic anatomy of women increases the likelihood of bladder infections because the passage between the bladder and the urethra is relatively short. This makes it easier for bacteria to enter the bladder. Bacteria may also get into the bladder by being pushed upward during sexual intercourse.

KEY POINTS

- Women are particularly prone to incontinence.
- Hormonal changes in pregnancy and menopause can cause problems.
- Physical damage to nerves and tissues may occur during childbirth.
- The pelvic anatomy of women increases the likelihood of bladder infections.

Finding out what's wrong

It is important to have your condition investigated if you suffer from episodes of involuntary urinary leakage. After a general examination at your doctor's office, you may be referred for specialized diagnostic tests at your local hospital.

GETTING HELP

If you are suffering from urinary incontinence, even if only slightly, and it is affecting the way in which you live, then you should ask for help. Your first step should be to make an appointment to see your primary care physician. He or she may be able to identify a cause of the incontinence, such as a urinary tract infection, and he or she may be able to administer the appropriate treatment. Your doctor may also order diagnostic testing; alternatively, you might be referred to a continence specialist physician or nurse for further evaluation and treatment of your problem.

SEEKING ADVICE
Anyone who suffers urinary incontinence severe enough to cause problems should consult her doctor.

INVESTIGATING THE PROBLEM

As we have seen, incontinence can have several different causes, and, before treatment can begin, the doctor will need to find out exactly what is causing your particular problem.

One of the first things that you will be tested for is a urinary tract infection because it is easily treated and can cause false results in later urodynamics tests.

The main aim of investigation is to find out if you have stress incontinence, which is caused by weakness of the bladder neck, or urge incontinence, which is caused by an unstable bladder. It may not be easy for the doctor to tell from your symptoms alone because these can be variable and it is possible to have both problems. If this is the case, treatment may be started and then the tests repeated to see if there has been any improvement.

Tests may also be performed to detect other rare causes of incontinence.

SIMPLE TESTS

The patient may be asked to fill in a five-day chart that records liquid intake and urine volume along with the frequency of urination. The chart is called frequency/volume diary and is a simple way to show quickly and accurately how the bladder usually functions. The diary may in itself indicate the cause of the problem. For example, someone developing diabetes will show increased liquid intake and increased frequency of urinating large volumes.

The diary may reveal inadequate fluid intake. This leads to highly concentrated urine that can irritate the bladder, producing symptoms of frequency and urgency. It can also predispose the person to urinary tract infections because the excretion of only small quantities of urine diminishes the body's natural defenses against bacteria entering the bladder.

Leakage can be measured by a pad test. A weighed sanitary napkin is worn for about an hour with a full bladder. During this time, the patient performs a series of basic exercises such as sitting down and standing up, walking up and down stairs, and washing the hands. The pad is then reweighed to calculate the volume of urine excreted.

URODYNAMICS

The standard tests that are performed to assess bladder function are collectively referred to as urodynamics tests. They measure the relationship between pressure and volume in the bladder and whether or not these are normal.

When urodynamics tests are performed, you have to go to the doctor's office or laboratory with a full bladder and urinate into a special toilet that measures the urinary flow rate. You are then examined and small pressure transducers, or detectors, are placed in the bladder and in the rectum. Although this can be embarrassing, it should not be painful.

The bladder is then filled through a catheter so that it reaches full capacity again within five minutes. During this period, the pressures from the two transducers are recorded. When the bladder is full again, the patient performs simple actions such as coughing and jumping to enable the doctor to see what happens to the pressures

FREQUENCY/VOLUME DIARY
One of the simplest means of testing your bladder function is a chart that records fluid intake, volume of urine, and frequency of urination.

and whether there is any leakage of urine. Finally, the patient empties her bladder into the special toilet with the pressure lines still in place for a "pressure flow plot" that allows an analysis to be made of bladder pressure during urination.

Although nobody likes the thought of these tests, they can usually be done relatively easily and with little embarrassment. The doctors and nurses who perform them are skilled in the techniques and try to make the tests as tolerable as possible.

In some hospitals, cystometry, the measurement of the pressure and volume of the bladder both when full and during emptying, may be used with X-ray imaging to examine the position of the bladder neck when leakage occurs during coughing. This test, known as video urodynamics, is of particular value in women who have had surgery or complicated problems.

The value of urodynamics testing is limited because it affords only a glimpse of the bladder's function during a relatively short period of about 20 minutes. However, in some hospitals the procedure can take up to four hours in order to allow the bladder to fill naturally, thereby replicating the actual circumstances that provoke incontinence.

IMAGING

There are two procedures that are commonly used to determine whether other parts of the urinary tract have been affected. These tests look for damage from infection or from the passage of urine the wrong way, up the ureter from the bladder to the kidney. They are also used to look for kidney stones.

The first test is called an intravenous urogram. This involves injecting dye into a vein in the arm that is then excreted through the kidneys. A series of X-rays are taken at timed intervals. The dye outlines the kidneys, ureters, and bladder, allowing the anatomy of the whole area to be examined.

The second method is an ultrasound scan, which can be used to examine the bladder and kidneys.

CYSTOSCOPY

A cystoscopy is performed to look at the inside of the bladder. A cystoscope is a narrow telescope that is passed into the bladder through the urethra.

There are two types of instruments: a flexible cystoscope, which is used under local anesthesia, and a rigid cystoscope, which requires general anesthesia. The advantage of the rigid cystoscope is that it allows samples of the lining of the bladder to be taken for analysis (see p.28).

NERVE TESTS

Occasionally, a test is performed to assess the nerve supply to the muscles of the bladder neck. This test, known as electromyography, involves the insertion of a needle electrode into the muscle of the urethra to measure electrical activity in the muscle.

How Cystoscopy Works

A cystoscope is a viewing instrument equipped with a lighting and lens system that enables a specialist to examine the internal wall of the bladder to check for any abnormalities.

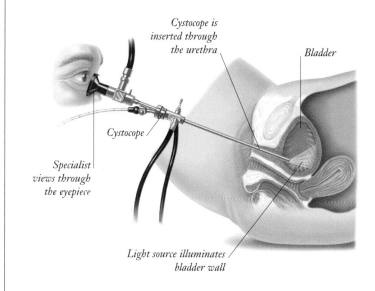

Cystocope is inserted through the urethra

Bladder

Cystocope

Specialist views through the eyepiece

Light source illuminates bladder wall

KEY POINTS

- Investigation is necessary to distinguish among stress incontinence, detrusor instability, and other causes of incontinence.
- A frequency/volume diary provides a simple way of showing how the bladder usually functions.
- Cystometry studies the pressure–volume relationship in the bladder.

Stress incontinence

The most common type of incontinence in women is stress incontinence, which accounts for about 40–50 percent of cases. Leakage occurs on coughing, sneezing, or exercising.

The most severely afflicted sufferers will leak with the slightest pressure on the bladder. Other women have a problem only during periods of extra exertion such as when exercising. The fear of leaking often discourages women from performing everyday activities such as aerobics or playing with grandchildren, and can be very restricting.

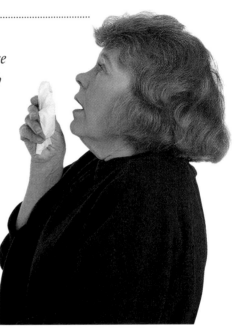

CREATING PRESSURE
Coughing or sneezing increases the pressure in the abdomen, and this in turn squeezes the bladder. If the urethra does not respond with equal pressure, leakage results.

Many women "manage" the condition by emptying their bladder regularly so that there is never enough urine in it to cause a serious problem. They are then able to avoid embarrassing wet patches by the use of a pad so that a small amount of leakage does not disrupt their lives. However, they may then find themselves having to visit every bathroom between any destination and home or making frequent trips to the bathroom at the office. Some women see their doctors because the

What Happens in Stress Incontinence

Stress incontinence occurs when the pressure within the bladder is raised without an equal rise in pressure at the bladder neck. Coughing, sneezing, or lifting a heavy weight causes increased intra-abdominal pressure on the bladder.

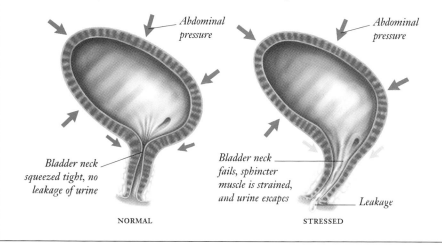

Abdominal pressure

Abdominal pressure

Bladder neck squeezed tight, no leakage of urine

Bladder neck fails, sphincter muscle is strained, and urine escapes

Leakage

NORMAL

STRESSED

situation is embarrassing. Others seek help because they are no longer able to cope with frequent changing of underwear or the prohibitive cost of pads.

WHAT CAUSES IT?

Stress incontinence commonly occurs as a result of a combination of weakening of the urethral sphincter or bladder neck, which seals the bladder between emptying, and a change in the position of the bladder neck.

There are many causes: hormonal changes during pregnancy and menopause, physical damage from childbirth, and straining when coughing or trying to have a bowel movement. Many women have a mixture of stress incontinence and urge incontinence.

As we explained earlier (pp.12–14), the urine inside the bladder exerts pressure on the bladder neck, which squeezes shut to resist the pressure and retain the urine inside the bladder. In order to stay dry, the sphincter muscles in the bladder neck must remain tightly closed when the pressure on the bladder from the outside increases with coughing, sneezing, or laughing.

Normally, the position of the bladder neck is such that any rise in pressure from coughing affects both bladder and urethra equally. If the bladder neck moves down from its normal position, the urethra is no longer compressed by the rise in pressure. In this case, the sphincter mechanism is put under more strain and urine escapes.

Teenage girls are prone to an embarrassing but self-limiting condition called giggle incontinence, in which they leak when they laugh but not at any other time. This condition is not properly understood but usually causes no major problems. Those who are affected can be reassured that it will disappear spontaneously without medical intervention.

WHAT IS THE TREATMENT?

There are a wide variety of treatments for stress incontinence, ranging from physical therapy to drug treatment to surgery.

To decide which is best, doctors will consider when the problem occurs, what is causing it, and your needs and preferences. For example, you may wish to reduce the leakage so that the problem can be managed with little disruption to your life, but you may not want to undergo surgery even though it could completely cure the condition.

NONSURGICAL TREATMENTS

• **Physical therapy** All affected women should have access to physical therapy. The type commonly employed for incontinence is called Kegel exercises or training (see opposite). This incorporates a series of exercises contracting the pelvic floor muscles, using repetition and endurance exercises designed to retrain and strengthen the muscles in the pelvic floor, leading to increased support of the bladder and urethra. Kegel exercises are both safe and effective with no side effects, but their efficacy greatly depends on the patient's motivation. They also require proper teaching and follow-up. They are ideal for women awaiting or unwilling to undergo an operation and for those medically unfit for surgery. Results of physical therapy are not immediate, and frequent regular exercise must be continued for at least 3–6 months to see any improvement. Maximal benefit is obtained only by correct long-term use.

Kegel exercises can be taught by doctors, nurses, or physical therapists. Normally, several visits to the office are needed to check that the contractions are being performed correctly and to help sustain your motivation. A worksheet to guide practice at home may be given.

Success rates vary, but with good instruction and strong motivation up to 70 percent of women may improve satisfactorily, although only 25 percent are completely cured.

• **Vaginal cones** Weighted vaginal cones (see p.34) can be used to strengthen the pelvic floor muscles and

Nonsurgical Treatments for Stress Incontinence

• Kegel exercises (physical therapy)
• Vaginal cones
• Biofeedback
• Drug therapy

How Kegel Exercises Work

If the pelvic floor muscles, which support the uterus, bowel, and bladder have become damaged or weakened, exercises that involve conscious tensing of these muscles can help strengthen them. This can help reduce stress incontinence.

CROSS-SECTION
SHOWN BELOW

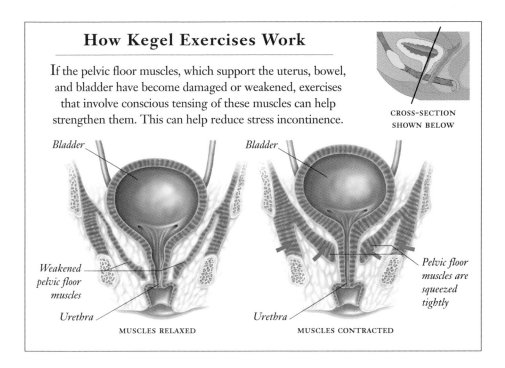

Bladder

Weakened pelvic floor muscles

Urethra

MUSCLES RELAXED

Bladder

Pelvic floor muscles are squeezed tightly

Urethra

MUSCLES CONTRACTED

may be particularly helpful in learning to identify the muscles of the pelvic floor. The cone is held in the vagina for increasing periods of time. When this can be done for two successive periods of 15 minutes, an identically sized but heavier cone is substituted. There are three to five different weights in a set of cones.

Cones are usually easier to learn to use than traditional Kegel exercises and require less follow-up supervision. However, Kegel exercises still form an essential part of treatment. Not all women are suited to the use of cones, and proper assessment is required first. If you have a large prolapse, for example, the cone can sit behind it without ever strengthening the pelvic floor muscles and in this case the use of cones is not beneficial.

33

- **Biofeedback** This technique, used to treat conditions such as high blood pressure, may also help women become more aware of their pelvic floor muscles.
- **Drug therapy** Medication is not usually helpful when stress incontinence is caused by weakness of the bladder neck. However, where there is evidence of estrogen deficiency, estrogen hormone treatment may be an important factor in increasing the success of other forms of treatment such as Kegel exercises. It works by improving the strength of tissues in the bladder, neck vagina, and pelvis, which weaken as a result of low estrogen levels. Estrogen treatment itself does not cure incontinence. Very occasionally, a medication called phenylpropanolamine, contained in some common cold

How Vaginal Cones Work

Weighted vaginal cones are sometimes used to strengthen the pelvic floor muscles. They are placed in the vagina for approximately 15 minutes.

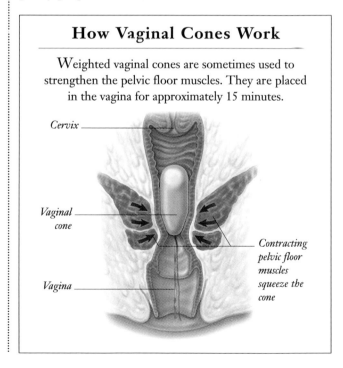

Cervix

Vaginal cone

Vagina

Contracting pelvic floor muscles squeeze the cone

remedies, is used. It artificially helps the muscle in the bladder neck contract to maintain a tight seal. Like estrogen, it is used in conjunction with other therapies to make up a complete treatment program. The use of this medication is less frequent, however, because Kegel exercises achieve better results and have no side effects.

SURGICAL TREATMENTS

To date, more than 250 different operations have been used to treat incontinence. A number of factors are taken into account when deciding which operation is best for a particular woman, including whether it is a first operation or repeat surgery, the local medical facilities, and the objectives of the patient. All surgery carries risk, and the more complex the operation, the greater the risk of complications.

> ### Surgical Treatments for Stress Incontinence
>
> - Bladder neck injections
> - Vaginal repairs with buttressing
> - Bladder neck suspensions
> - Colposuspensions
> - Sling procedures

There may thus be a trade-off when a simpler procedure is preferred because it is easier and shorter even though the success rate may be lower. Simpler procedures also have shorter recovery periods.

Incontinence surgery is divided into five classes. Some operations require the surgeon to open up the abdominal cavity. In others, the procedure can be performed through the vagina. Abdominal procedures have higher success rates than the other types of operations, but they tend to involve a longer recovery period. These operations are considered more complex because they require an incision on the abdominal wall along the bikini line.

- **Bladder neck injections** The simplest type of procedure involves injecting one of a number of bulking agents into the bladder neck. The most commonly used substances are tiny silicone particles and collagen. Some surgeons undertake this as an outpatient procedure performed under local or regional anesthesia, but more commonly it is performed under general anesthesia.

This type of operation aims to increase the resistance at the bladder neck by bringing its edges together so that urine cannot leak out easily. It has a relatively low absolute cure rate, although it usually leads to some improvement. It is relatively easy to repeat if necessary and generally does not cause significant scarring.

Occasionally, women have problems emptying their bladders after this type of operation, but this is usually transient, and most women tolerate the injection well with little discomfort.

- **Vaginal repair** The aim of vaginal repair is to reposition the bladder and urethra by pushing them up. This type of operation can be performed to repair a prolapse, in which the uterus has moved down into the vagina, or to elevate the bladder neck in order to restore continence. The vagina and the pelvic muscles are tightened up, restoring the bladder to its proper position.

Vaginal repair is a simple procedure, and patients recover rapidly. It is often initially successful and is currently the second most common type of operation performed for stress incontinence. However, recent studies have cast doubt on its long-term success rate.

- **Bladder neck suspensions** In these operations, the bladder neck is lifted by passing two sutures on each side of it and securing them above the muscle in the abdominal wall. It is a relatively straightforward procedure that is easy to perform and has low complication rates. After bladder neck suspensions, some women occasionally have problems urinating. If the bladder neck has been lifted too far, the bladder neck may become partially obstructed, although this is not usually a permanent problem.

• **Colposuspension** The term "colposuspension" means "supporting the vagina." This is achieved by carefully dissecting the bladder neck free of its attachments and passing stitches through the supporting structures at the sides. These stitches are then tied to the ligament or to the bone itself on the inside of the pelvis. The operation is performed through an abdominal incision along the bikini line and therefore requires a longer recovery period than the other surgical procedures.

• **Sling procedures** These operations, which can be performed as an abdominal or a vaginal procedure, pass a sling under the urethra and stitch it to the abdominal wall. A wide variety of materials are used for the sling, from autografts (strips of material removed from another part of the body such as the rectus sheath) to artificial materials such as Teflon and Goretex tape. A promising new type of sling operation using tension-free vaginal tape is undergoing clinical trials. It offers the advantages of a sling but is a vaginal operation that can be performed as an outpatient procedure.

One of the most common side effects of this type of surgery for stress incontinence is transient obstruction, in which there is difficulty emptying the bladder. In the short term, this may occur in as many as 20 percent of those who have the operation. For most, however, it is no more than a minor setback, and, over a longer period of time, bladder function returns to normal. Simple retraining in emptying the bladder may help, such as sitting with the legs farther apart and leaning forward.

Some women, however, require a longer period of catheterization to rest the bladder, usually around 10–14 days. Occasionally, women need to be taught how to catheterize themselves if voiding difficulties persist. This can usually be achieved easily and should be no more troublesome than having to change a tampon. Most women agree that the inconvenience of having to catheterize is preferable to the embarrassment caused by incontinence. Sometimes it is possible to predict who is at risk of voiding difficulties before surgery is performed. In these cases, self-catheterization

How Bladder Neck Suspension Works

In this straightforward surgical procedure, sutures are passed from behind the bladder on each side of the bladder neck and then secured above the muscle in the abdominal wall, raising the bladder neck.

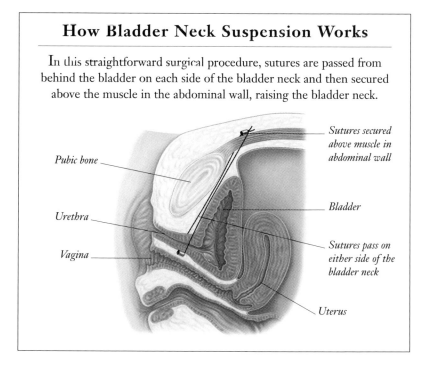

Pubic bone

Urethra

Vagina

Sutures secured above muscle in abdominal wall

Bladder

Sutures pass on either side of the bladder neck

Uterus

may be taught beforehand (see pp.56–57). The other complication of these operations is the development of irritating symptoms such as frequency and urgency. This occurs in about 10 percent of women. Nobody understands the reason for the occurrence of these symptoms, and it is usually unpredictable.

KEY POINTS

- Stress incontinence accounts for 40–50 percent of women with incontinence problems.
- It can be caused by anything that weakens the bladder neck support and causes its position to drop.
- Kegel exercises can help up to 75 percent of all women.
- There is a wide range of surgical operations to treat the condition.

Urge incontinence

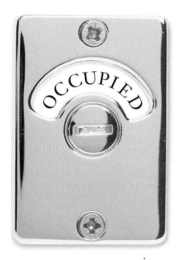

The second most common type of incontinence is urge incontinence. Urgency is the sudden and uncontrollable need to urinate. If a toilet is not reached in time, there may be leakage. Occasional urgency is normal, but it is a problem if you feel that the symptoms are affecting your lifestyle or if you have recurrent infections.

NO TIME TO SPARE
Urge incontinence can make a trip to the toilet imperative and can lead to leakage if there is any delay.

In most cases, urge incontinence results from an instability of the muscle in the bladder wall, the detrusor muscle. The condition is known as detrusor instability. The detrusor muscle contracts to force urine out through the bladder neck during urination. Normally this muscle does not contract before the time is appropriate. However, if the muscle is unstable or overactive, it may contract involuntarily, resulting in the sensation of urgency and the need to urinate more often than normal.

Incontinence can result from instability of the detrusor muscle if the bladder neck is weak or if it is opened by the force of the contraction. The problem tends to wax and wane and is often worse during the colder winter months.

The involuntary contractions can be triggered by a variety of things. Coughing is one of them, and therefore people with detrusor instability can have the symptoms of stress incontinence because they leak when they cough. A variety of triggers such as the sight and sound of running water can also act as a trigger for incontinence. The fuller the bladder, the more likely it is that involuntary contractions will occur.

Urge Incontinence

Urge incontinence normally occurs when the detrusor muscle is unstable or overactive. Also known as detrusor instability, this condition causes a sensation of urgency or the need to urinate frequently.

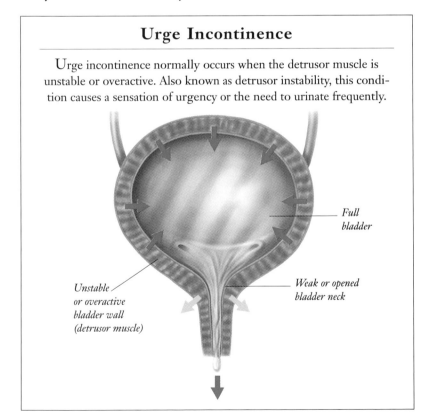

Full bladder

Unstable or overactive bladder wall (detrusor muscle)

Weak or opened bladder neck

Detrusor instability with involuntary contractions is known as motor urgency.

The other major type of urgency is sensory urgency, in which the bladder feels very uncomfortable but there is no actual leaking. The differentiation of these two problems – motor urgency and sensory urgency – requires a variety of urodynamics tests (see pp.25–26), although there are other features that may suggest what the problem might be.

THE CAUSES

In most cases, the cause of urge incontinence is not known. Detrusor instability may be related to loss of normal control of the bladder-emptying reflex or to overactivity of one of the nerves supplying the bladder. Nerve damage and neurological conditions such as stroke and multiple sclerosis can cause the bladder to contract in an unstable way. If the instability has a known neurological cause, the condition is known as detrusor hyperreflexia.

In many cases, people who develop the condition have a history of bed-wetting as children or have always had a "weak bladder." This may be a result of poor bladder training in childhood. Quite often, other members of the family have had problems as well.

Women who have had incontinence surgery may also be prone to the condition. The surgery may have

BED-WETTING
Children who have incomplete bladder control and continue to wet the bed can suffer from urge incontinence later in life.

partially blocked the bladder neck to stop leakage. The bladder's response is to cause the muscle to thicken, and in some cases the normal control mechanism is lost, resulting in an unstable bladder.

TREATMENT OPTIONS

Treatment of detrusor instability is directed at developing control of bladder contraction. This may be achieved by behavioral therapy or by the use of medication. Both of these treatment approaches address the symptoms rather than the cause of the problem, and neither offers a cure.

BEHAVIORAL THERAPY

Behavioral therapy works by retraining the brain to control the bladder more effectively, in particular by suppressing the involuntary contractions that cause urge incontinence.

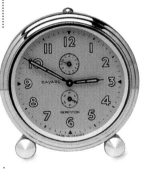

BY THE CLOCK
A strict regime of urinating at set times helps many women overcome their urge incontinence. An alarm clock can also help cure children of bed-wetting.

The mainstay of behavioral therapy is bladder drill. First the bladder is emptied. An interval is then set, usually an hour, during which the woman is not allowed to use the toilet, even if this causes leaking. After the hour has passed the woman must urinate. This is then repeated so that a pattern of regular voiding is established. The interval is slowly increased as each target is repeatedly met. The aim is to urinate once every three hours.

Bladder drill has been shown to be highly effective in treating urge incontinence when taught to patients in the hospital, with up to 85 percent of women showing dramatic improvement. It does, however, require a very high level of motivation and commitment in the patient, along with encouragement from the hospital staff.

Consequently, there is a very high relapse rate after discharge, when patients have resumed a normal lifestyle that may not always allow for a strict toilet regimen. There is usually less encouragement and support outside the hospital, although bladder drill is also taught and supervised in the community by doctors and office nurses. Despite the problems in maintaining progress, bladder drill remains an important tool in the management of an unstable bladder.

Biofeedback (see p.34) can be used to help with bladder drill. Electrical sensors are used to detect bladder activity,

Control of the Bladder

When the bladder is under proper control, the pressure within the full bladder is contained by the contraction of sphincter muscles in the bladder neck and the urethra. These are then consciously relaxed to allow the urine to flow out.

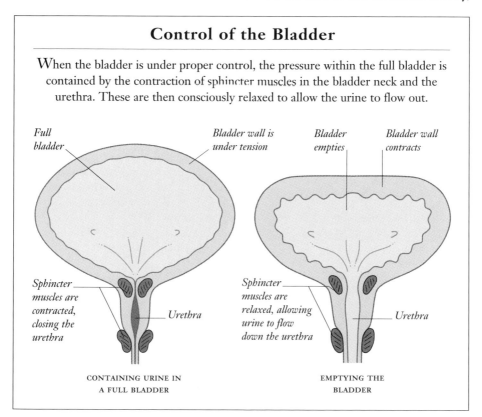

Full bladder

Bladder wall is under tension

Bladder empties

Bladder wall contracts

Sphincter muscles are contracted, closing the urethra

Urethra

Sphincter muscles are relaxed, allowing urine to flow down the urethra

Urethra

CONTAINING URINE IN
A FULL BLADDER

EMPTYING THE
BLADDER

which helps patients identify the sensation of bladder contraction so that they can learn to suppress it.

The principle of bladder drill can be applied to bed-wetting. In this case, it involves knowing when the bed-wetting occurs and setting an alarm clock to ring beforehand. When incontinence is regularly avoided, the interval can be gradually increased.

DRUG TREATMENTS

The medications that are most commonly used in the treatment of an unstable bladder are the anticholinergic drugs. These preparations act by blocking the impulses between the nerves that control the bladder and the bladder muscle itself. In this way, the response of the muscle to stimulation is suppressed. Since these drugs treat the symptoms rather than the cause of the problem, drug treatment may need to be continued indefinitely. Generally, the first medication tried is oxybutynin.

The major problems with anticholinergic medications are side effects in parts of the body other than the bladder. The most common are dry mouth, blurry vision, constipation, heartburn, palpitations, and, if the drug acts too effectively, difficulty urinating. They cannot be used if you have glaucoma, and some people find that the pills make them drowsy or tired. Even so, although most people have some side effects (and they must be anticipated to some extent if the medication is to be successful), the benefits make it worthwhile.

If the side effects are pronounced, a tricyclic anti-depressant (amitriptyline or imipramine) may be used

DISTURBED NIGHTS
Some people who find themselves regularly waking in the night because of the need to urinate can be helped by desmopressin, which reduces the production of urine.

45

instead. These medications also have anticholinergic effects but they have less severe side effects. The newer anticholinergic medications and longer-acting forms of traditional anticholinergics such as tolterodine have fewer side effects.

Another approach to managing the condition is the use of an artificial hormone called desmopressin. This hormone signals to the kidneys to decrease urine production, thereby reducing the rate of bladder filling. This drug is particularly helpful at night, when urine production should be naturally reduced, allowing uninterrupted sleep. The problem with this type of treatment is that it cannot be used continually; if the kidneys produce less urine at night, they must compensate and produce more during the day. Desmopressin is therefore used predominantly in children who wet the bed and in adults whose symptoms are worst at night. It is not usually given to people who may be at risk if they retain extra fluid, for example, people with high blood pressure or heart problems.

Estrogens may also be used as part of a management strategy to prevent the dryness and thinning of the vaginal lining that normally develop after menopause.

CHANGES IN DIET AND LIFESTYLE

Smoking is known to irritate the bladder and make an unstable bladder worse. Caffeine and alcohol have a doubly bad effect because they stimulate not only the bladder but also the kidneys to produce more urine. Therefore, the instability of the bladder is increased while it must also handle a greater volume of urine.

Side Effects of Anticholinergics

- Blurry vision
- Dry mouth
- Constipation
- Urinary retention
- Heartburn
- Palpitations

Caffeine is found not only in coffee but also in tea and some sodas, all of which can worsen symptoms.

For some people, simple adjustments in their living arrangements may be sufficient. For example, a woman with reduced mobility may leak in the morning because her bladder is full and she cannot walk to the bathroom without significant effort. Having a commode by the bed may solve her problem.

KEY POINTS

- Urge incontinence results from instability of the muscle in the bladder wall.
- In most cases, the cause is unknown.
- Treatment entails either behavioral therapy or medication.
- These treatments address symptoms but do not offer a cure.
- Changes in diet and lifestyle may help.

Problems in emptying the bladder

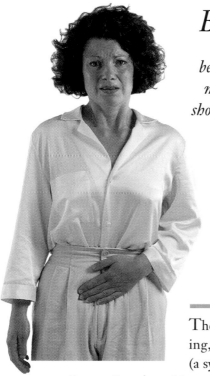

*B*roadly speaking, problems in emptying
the bladder, known as voiding, can
be divided into two groups. If the bladder
muscle is weak or does not contract as it
should, the bladder will not empty properly.
Or, if the bladder neck cannot relax
or is scarred, it will be difficult for
the bladder muscle to force urine
past it. In both cases, the bladder
may not empty completely. These
processes can occur independently
or simultaneously.

STOMACH PAIN
*Discomfort just above the
pelvic bone may be due to an
inflammation of the bladder
known as cystitis.*

SYMPTOMS

The symptoms include burning pain on urinating, difficulty emptying the bladder completely
(a symptom that is often associated with prostate
problems in men), and leaking.

RECURRENT CYSTITIS

Recurrent cystitis is a common complaint among
women who may have an underlying difficulty emptying the bladder. This difficulty impairs the normal

Effects of Cystitis on the Bladder

Cystitis is an inflammation of the inside of the bladder, usually due to a bacterial infection. Bacteria that are harmless in the bowel can cause cystitis if they get into the urinary tract.

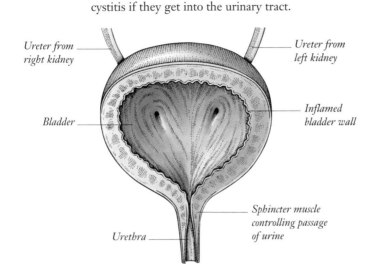

Ureter from right kidney

Ureter from left kidney

Bladder

Inflamed bladder wall

Sphincter muscle controlling passage of urine

Urethra

mechanisms that protect against bladder infection. Bacteria are normally washed away from the bladder and the area outside the urethra during voiding. If the bladder is not emptying properly, the bacteria will stay there longer and will therefore be more likely to cause infection.

HESITANCY

The symptom of hesitancy involves the sensation of wanting to void and a delay between trying to and actually urinating. In an extreme form, hesitancy leads to strangury, which is gradual voiding accompanied by pain. This

Symptoms of Voiding Difficulties

- Recurrent infections
- Hesitancy
- Urgency and frequency
- Retention
- Overflow incontinence
- Bladder pain

condition is more common in men, in whom it is associated with prostatism.

URGENCY AND FREQUENCY

If the bladder does not empty properly, its capacity is reduced, which may result in increased frequency of urination and nocturia (getting up at night more often than normal to urinate). Urgency, the sudden and uncontrollable need to urinate, may also be a problem.

RETENTION

Retention is a condition in which the bladder cannot empty. If this occurs suddenly, it is usually very painful and requires immediate action to prevent damage to the bladder as a result of prolonged overfilling.

Chronic retention is usually painless. This type of retention occurs because the bladder outlet gradually becomes obstructed, for example, as the result of a fibroid pressing on the urethra or because the bladder is increasingly unable to create enough muscle power to enable emptying.

The first step in the treatment of retention is to drain the bladder with a catheter. The doctor may then arrange for tests to determine the cause of the condition, such as an ultrasound scan to check for a mass pressing on the bladder as well as to measure the volume of urine remaining in the bladder.

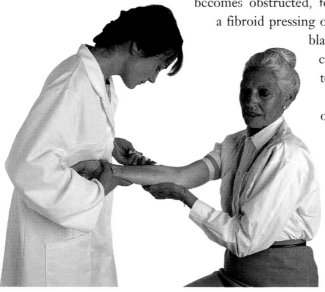

HAVING A BLOOD TEST
When retention is a problem, a sample of blood may be taken to check whether damage has been caused to the kidneys.

A blood test may be ordered to check that the kidneys have not been damaged by the pressure that has been exerted on them by the full bladder. Urodynamics testing (see pp.25–26) is also used to evaluate bladder function.

OVERFLOW INCONTINENCE

When the bladder is unable to empty because of an obstruction or decreased ability to contract, the pressure inside it will eventually build up so much that urine leaks "over the top." This condition is known as overflow incontinence. In some cases, there may be an almost continuous leakage of urine (dribble incontinence).

Overflow incontinence is most often seen in men who are experiencing prostate problems, but it can also occur in women, particularly if there is pressure on the bladder from a large uterine fibroid. Overflow incontinence can also occur in association with other medical problems, such as multiple sclerosis, in which bladder coordination is gradually lost. In these cases, the bladder contracts to empty but at the same time the urethral sphincter contracts to prevent the bladder from emptying (see pp.12–16). Dribble incontinence also may be caused by fistulas (see pp.70–71).

BLADDER PAIN

Bladder pain caused by voiding difficulties usually results from an intense need to empty the bladder, called

Causes of Urinary Retention and Voiding Difficulties

- Drugs
- Nerve injury/neurological problems
- Childbirth
- Epidural anesthesia
- Fibroids or pelvic masses
- Constipation
- Surgery
- Narrowing of the urethra
- Prolapse

urgency. The pain is normally "suprapubic," just above the pelvic bone.

Infections are often associated with this intense urgency. Classically, however, infections also cause a burning pain during urination. In severe cases, a dull ache may remain after voiding.

CAUSES OF VOIDING PROBLEMS

There are many possible reasons for a person to experience problems with voiding, including drugs, nerve damage, childbirth, fibroids, and pelvic surgery.

DRUGS

Medications such as antidepressants can suppress the bladder's ability to contract. If the bladder function is already relatively weak, this can tip the balance between being able to empty and going into retention.

NERVE DAMAGE

Damage to the nerves that supply the bladder can alter the ability of the bladder muscle to contract. Consequently, a chronic or severe back problem (for example, a slipped disk) can trigger difficulties.

CHILDBIRTH

Urinary retention commonly results from childbirth, particularly after epidural anesthesia, which decreases bladder nerve function. In women who have had epidural anesthesia, an indwelling catheter is inserted to protect the bladder until normal sensation returns after about

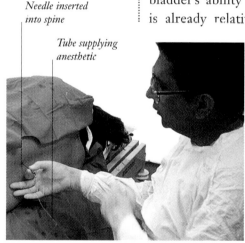

Needle inserted into spine

Tube supplying anesthetic

EPIDURAL ANESTHESIA
When epidural anesthesia is given to reduce the pain of childbirth, the loss of sensation can produce temporary incontinence.

12 hours. There is also an increased risk after a forceps delivery or when there is marked trauma to the perineum and vagina that may make urination painful. Consequently, the patient avoids urinating and eventually becomes unable to void.

FIBROIDS

Fibroids are a common gynecological cause of difficulties emptying the bladder. Fibroids are benign tumors that grow in the womb. If the fibroids cause an external obstruction to the bladder neck, it becomes increasingly difficult to empty the bladder. As the fibroids grow, the problem increases until the woman goes into urinary retention. Any other lump or mass occurring in the pelvis, such as fecal impaction, can cause similar problems.

SURGERY

One of the most common causes of temporary voiding difficulties is pelvic surgery, and incontinence surgery in particular. When the bladder neck is lifted to reposition it, an element of obstruction can be created. If the pressure of the contraction of the bladder muscle cannot overcome this, there will be difficulties emptying the bladder. Most women who have had a colposuspension, for example, will notice that they void at a slower rate after surgery.

Postoperative voiding difficulties can be divided into short-term and long-term problems. About 20 percent of women have minor voiding dysfunction that clears up with careful catheter management. Of these, about one percent will experience chronic problems that require long-term treatment.

The most successful way to manage the problem is self-catheterization, which allows the woman to control her symptoms and gives her the freedom to lead a normal life (see pp.56–57).

STRICTURES IN THE URETHRA

Stricture or narrowing of the urethra is now relatively uncommon in women. It can occur if trauma or an infection damages the lining of the urethra, which then heals with scarring. Strictures cause voiding difficulties by reducing the size of the urethra and thereby causing outflow obstruction. Urethral strictures require an operation either to dilate or to cut the narrowing, but the condition needs to be carefully assessed before treatment to check that there are no other problems and to insure that treatment will not further damage the urethra. Strictures often recur and sometimes require repeated treatment.

BLADDER PROLAPSE

Bladder prolapse can cause problems with voiding by kinking the urethra and thereby obstructing it. This is like kinking a hose to prevent water from flowing out. Correction of the prolapse restores the bladder neck to the normal position, allowing normal voiding. Prolapse and incontinence often coexist because the damage that causes prolapse also leads to stress incontinence.

WEAK DETRUSOR MUSCLE

The detrusor muscle gets weaker with age and contracts less efficiently. The bladder wall also becomes stiffer. As a result, the bladder functions less well. These are normal effects of aging that account for the longer time elderly people take to empty their bladders as well as their increased frequency of urination.

Occasionally, the nerves to the bladder stop working properly, which prevents the detrusor muscle from contracting properly. Nerve damage to the bladder occurs after urinary retention or as a result of nerve damage from diabetes, multiple sclerosis, or stroke.

This may not in itself always lead to a problem because part of voiding is relaxation of the pelvic floor, which may be enough on its own to allow emptying. Usually, however, women require active force to empty their bladders.

INVESTIGATIONS AND TESTS

Voiding difficulties require thorough investigation with urodynamics testing (see pp.25–26). If there is pain in the flanks or there have been serious kidney infections, tests will be performed to check that urine does not flow the wrong way, up the ureter from the bladder to the kidneys. A test to check the pressure in the urethra, called a urethral pressure profile, may also be performed.

In many cases, particularly if there is a history of infection, a cystoscopy may be performed (see pp.27–28). This allows the doctor to inspect the inside of the bladder through an endoscope, under local or general anesthesia, and allows small biopsy samples to be taken from the bladder for analysis.

TREATMENT OPTIONS

Often mild degrees of difficulty can be managed with simple measures. When sitting on the toilet, make sure your knees are apart rather than together. Leaning forward or even standing slightly may alter the angle of the bladder neck enough to allow better emptying. Waiting for two minutes after the initial voiding and then trying again may also help. This is known as the double-void technique. More severe symptoms may require medical treatment.

There are three approaches to the treatment of difficulties voiding:

● **Try to increase the force of bladder contractions** This can be achieved in some cases with bethanechol, a drug that stimulates the nerve fibers controlling the contraction of the bladder muscle. This may be effective if there are no signs of obstruction at the bladder neck or urethra.

● **Try to reduce outflow obstruction** This method is used if there is a specific site of obstruction in the urethra, such as a stricture, or if narrowing has been demonstrated during the investigation outlined on page 55.

● **Use a catheter** Catheters can either be used occasionally or can remain in place long-term.

Occasional self-catheterization, when it is properly taught to a healthy individual with normal dexterity, is the best option. It allows the freedom to control your symptoms with little more inconvenience than that involved in changing a tampon.

CATHETERIZATION

A catheter is a soft, flexible tube that is thinner than a pencil and has a rounded end. When passed up the urethra into the bladder, it allows all the urine to flow out without muscular effort.

Although the thought of having to catheterize is initially upsetting to most women, when they have

How a Catheter Works

Catheterization may be an effective way of dealing with voiding difficulties. A catheter is inserted through the ureter into the bladder and allows urine to pass without effort. It is held in place by a small balloon at its upper end.

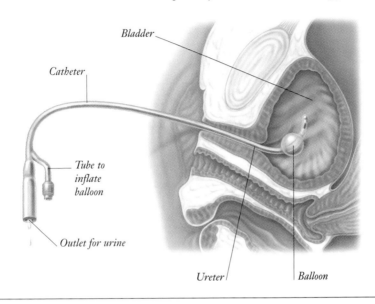

Bladder

Catheter

Tube to inflate balloon

Outlet for urine

Ureter

Balloon

learned the technique and are confident, they find it far easier than expected. The technique requires a basic understanding of pelvic anatomy and instruction in identifying the urethra. Initially, a mirror is helpful, but in time most women manage without one.

With practice, inserting a catheter through the urethra is normally not painful. The number of times you need to catheterize depends on how your bladder functions. If the catheter is to be left in place long-term, it will be retained by a balloon inflated within the bladder (see box above).

KEY POINTS

- Difficulties emptying the bladder may cause a variety of symptoms.
- Retention can be caused by drugs, nerve damage, childbirth, fibroids, or pelvic surgery.
- Simple measures may be sufficient to deal with mild cases.
- Self-catheterization may be an effective way of managing the problem if simpler methods have not been effective.

Urinary tract infections

The urinary tract is made up of the kidneys, ureters, bladder, and urethra. Infection of any of these organs can spread to the others.

The symptoms of urinary tract infections may differ widely. Some women have no symptoms at all, and the infection remains hidden until it causes kidney failure. Other women experience pain, urinary frequency, and burning, burning, and may have blood in their urine. If a woman experiences a urinary infection at least three times per year, she is said to have recurrent infections.

WHAT CAUSES INFECTIONS?

Bacteria are small organisms that are found everywhere. Normally they do not cause an infection when they are in their usual habitat, and it is not unusual to find bacteria in a healthy woman's bladder. However, if the balance of bacteria changes, there may be overgrowth of one type that can cause damage resulting in an infection. Cystitis is an inflammation of the bladder that can result from infection. The female urethra

DRINKING PLENTY
Some women claim that drinking plenty of water will clear up an infection, but the effect may be due to the extra liquid diluting the urine.

(the passage between the bladder and the outside) is relatively short, which allows easy access to the bladder for bacteria that are normally found around the vagina and perineum (the area between the vagina and the anus). Quite often, these bacteria are the same as those found in the bowel. When the bladder empties, it washes them out, and, as the urine leaves the body, it cleans the area just outside the urethra.

Difficulty emptying the bladder is a major cause of infection. If the bladder does not empty completely, these bacteria stay in it and can start to multiply. If the bacteria increase in number, they can then damage the lining of the bladder and produce inflammation. This in turn causes the symptoms of burning and frequency that are characteristic of cystitis.

Another important factor in infection is sexual intercourse. During intercourse, the bacteria that are normally present outside the urethra can be pushed into it and spread up into the bladder. This is known as auto- or self-infection. In addition, other types of bacteria can be introduced from the man. Sexual intercourse can also cause small abrasions that can give the bacteria a stronger foothold from which to colonize the bladder.

There are simple measures that can be used to avoid infections associated with sexual intercourse. Emptying the bladder completely soon after sex may help wash out the bacteria. In order to gain the full protective effect, however, the bladder must first be at least comfortably full. Emptying only a small drop out of the bladder will not wash away all the bacteria.

You should also consider the type of contraceptive method that you use. In about 10 percent of all women, urinary infections can occur as a result of using the diaphragm and spermicide, and in some cases changing to condom use will prevent infections. Some women are allergic to the most widely used spermicide, nonoxynol-9.

Simple hygienic measures may also help decrease the growth of bacteria on the outside of the vagina. One such measure is to wipe from the vagina toward the anus after using the toilet. Douching is unwise because it usually removes the natural, helpful bacteria, allowing more harmful bowel bacteria to colonize, and maactually increase the risk of infection. The vagina is a self-cleaning organ and does not require special detergents or perfumes.

Kidney and bladder stones are another rare cause of infections. If bacteria infect a stone, it is almost impossible to clear the infection. In these cases, the stone must be removed. Infections are also more common during pregnancy (see p.18).

INVESTIGATING AN INFECTION

When you see your doctor because you have the symptoms of a urinary infection, the doctor may treat the problem without diagnosing its cause through urinalysis or a culture. However, if you have unusual or recurrent symptoms, or signs of an upper urinary tract infection such as fever or low back pain, then urine samples will be taken to determine the types of bacteria that are causing the infection. The urine sample must be a midstream specimen. This is collected by starting to empty the bladder and, when the stream is estab- lished, catching a sample in a sterile container. The reason for discarding the first part of the stream is that it can be contaminated by bacteria that are present on the skin and in the urethra. The midstream urine sample should yield a representative specimen from inside the bladder. Analysis of the urine sample will indicate whether you are developing different urine infections or recurrence of the same one that is not being adequately treated.

Women who have demonstrated recurrent bladder infections require further investigation (see Investigating the problem, pp.24–28) to exclude other causes of infection, such as chronic kidney infection. A frequency/volume diary may provide important information regarding the behavior of your bladder. Urodynamics testing and cystoscopy are routinely used to evaluate bladder function and to visualize the interior of the bladder.

TREATING AN INFECTION

A mild infection may disappear on its own, requiring only the treatment described below. Many women believe that drinking a lot of water cures a urinary infection. It is more likely that the water alleviates the symptoms by keeping the urine diluted while the bladder is sore, allowing the body's natural defenses to clear up the infection. Cranberry juice is also commonly suggested as a treatment for cystitis. It may help reduce the acidity of urine, thereby making voiding less painful.

Established infections require adequate treatment with an appropriate antibiotic. Often doctors treat uncomplicated urinary infections empirically, which means that they prescribe an antibiotic likely to cure the infection without waiting for test results.

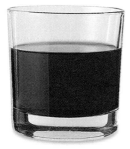

CRANBERRY JUICE
Some drinks, such as cranberry juice, may reduce the acidity of urine, making urination less painful.

Remember that, even though an antibiotic does not work on one occasion, it may work subsequently.

After excluding any underlying cause of the recurrent infections, there are two treatment options. The first approach is to prescribe an indefinite course of low-dose antibiotics, used at night in an attempt to keep the bladder sterile and prevent an infection. The second approach is to treat only when necessary.

If symptoms occur only after intercourse, an anti-biotic can be taken either before or immediately after-ward. Alternatively, most women who have recurrent cystitis know when symptoms are going to develop up to 12 hours beforehand. In this case, a single dose of an antibiotic often eliminates the symptoms. If they persist, additional antibiotics can be taken. Symptoms lasting longer than 24 hours usually indicate that the infection is resistant to the antibiotic.

Very occasionally, the infections are caused by "atypical" bacteria, such as ureaplasma and mycoplasma. Diagnosis of these infections usually requires special laboratory tests on the urine. These infections may require antibiotic treatment for about three months.

INTERSTITIAL CYSTITIS

Interstitial cystitis is a rarely diagnosed inflammatory condition of the bladder, the cause of which is unclear. It causes bladder pain and mimics cystitis caused by an infection. This type of cystitis often causes frequency and urgency and can cause the bladder lining to bleed, leading to blood in the urine. It can also cause changes in the bladder's capacity and increased bladder sensi-tivity. A biopsy or sample of the bladder wall is required and, if interstitial cystitis is present, will show an increase in inflammatory cells, particularly mast cells (a type of immune cell).

Interstitial cystitis occurs almost exclusively in women, raising the question of whether there is a hormonal influence. Up to 95 percent of affected women are white, and symptoms start after the age of 20. This is around the age at which many women become sexually active, which makes it more difficult to distinguish interstitial cystitis from recurrent infections.

Although the cause of interstitial cystitis is still unknown, its effects are now beginning to be understood. The bladder wall becomes inflamed and thickens. This may be a direct result of an infection or may be caused by the action of the body's defense mechanisms against the cells of the bladder. These two possible mechanisms have led to most approaches to treatment.

TREATING INTERSTITIAL CYSTITIS

Common treatments include a variety of drugs. Antibiotics may be given for at least three months to keep the bladder free of any infection and to give the bladder wall a chance to heal and recover. Alternatively, bladder antiseptics taken orally can be used to try to create an environment conducive to healing. Drugs known to reduce inflammation can be used, and simple medications such as aspirin and other analgesics may help. A greater anti-inflammatory effect is achieved with steroids such as prednisone.

Another anti-inflammatory treatment employs antihistamines, more commonly used in the treatment of allergic rhinitis (hay fever) and stomach ulcers. The mast cells in the bladder wall release histamine, which is involved in causing inflammation. Antihistamines

reduce this effect and consequently may alleviate the
the symptoms.

Many other medications, such as antidepressants,
anticholinergics, and calcium antagonists, have been
suggested for interstitial cystitis. Unfortunately, the
causes of interstitial cystitis have not been identified,
and therefore medication can treat only the symptoms.

There are some lifestyle changes that appear to help.
These are based on the identification of trigger factors,
such as caffeine. Avoidance of these substances can
often be as effective as medication.

KEY POINTS

- Recurrent urinary tract infections are often related
  to sexual intercourse or to difficulties in emptying
  the bladder.
- Simple hygienic measures can help.
- Treatment of established infection requires antibiotics.
- Interstitial cystitis is a rare type of cystitis and may be
  confused with recurrent infection.

Other problems associated with incontinence

When a doctor sees a patient with incontinence for the first time, he or she will consider other aspects of the patient's health because other conditions can be associated with incontinence.

FINDING OUT MORE
Your doctor should investigate other possible associated conditions, such as fibroids, when treating you for incontinence.

MENSTRUAL PERIODS AND FIBROIDS

You will be asked about your menstrual periods because, if they are heavy and painful, you may have fibroids. These are benign tumors that grow in the uterus wall. They are very common and usually do not cause urinary problems. However, if fibroids cause distortion of the pelvic organs they can interfere with bladder anatomy

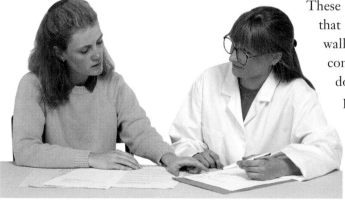

and function. In particular, fibroids can increase abdominal pressure and contribute to displacement of the bladder neck, which is associated with incontinence. If you are likely to need surgery for incontinence, it may be a good time to see whether the fibroids also need treatment.

PROLAPSE

Prolapse is the movement of the vaginal wall from its normal position along with the bladder, bowel, or uterus. It is caused by damage to the ligaments in the pelvis. These ligaments act as supports for the uterus and the muscle layers that lie over the bowel and bladder. The most common causes of prolapse are childbearing and conditions that cause chronic straining, such as

Uterine Prolapse

A prolapsed uterus occurs when the ligaments in the pelvis that hold the uterus in position are stretched in pregnancy or are weakened after menopause, causing the uterus to fall down into the vagina.

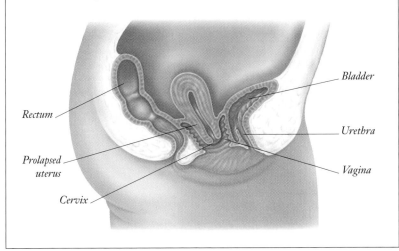

Rectum

Prolapsed uterus

Cervix

Bladder

Urethra

Vagina

constipation, smoker's cough, and obesity. There are several types of prolapse, which are graded according to severity. A cystocele is a prolapse of the front wall of the vagina along with the bladder. Uterine prolapse refers to the uterus coming down through the vagina. A rectocele is a prolapse of the back wall of the vagina with the bowel coming down behind it.

Prolapse may occur on its own or in conjunction with other symptoms, such as incontinence and difficulty with bowel movements. Common complaints include the feeling of "something coming down" and discomfort or pain during sexual intercourse.

Treatment of prolapse is dependent on several factors, including your own wishes and the degree to which the prolapse interferes with your life. The best results are usually obtained with surgery to place the organs back into their proper positions, but this is not always the most appropriate treatment. You may not have completed your family, and another childbirth could cause the prolapse to recur. Or you may not be well enough or willing to undergo surgery. Sometimes silicone rings called pessaries can be placed in the vagina. If they eliminate symptoms, they can be used continuously, and only require changing every six months. A major drawback is that the pessary sits in the vagina, making sexual intercourse difficult.

DIABETES

Diabetes may affect the bladder in many ways, from causing frequency as a result of excessive drinking to damaging the nerve supply to the bladder. In the latter case, diabetes can cause detrusor instability or difficulties emptying the bladder or both, depending on the exact effect of the diabetes on the nerves. Therefore, it is important to be tested for diabetes if you have symptoms such as excessive thirst, frequency, and weight loss, or if there is a history of diabetes in your family.

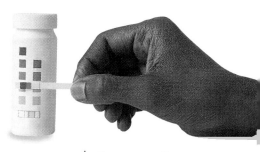

CHECKING FOR DIABETES
If you suspect that you are suffering from diabetes, make sure that you have appropriate blood and urine tests to check your glucose levels.

BOWEL PROBLEMS

Many women who have bladder symptoms, particularly women with an unstable bladder, also suffer from bowel symptoms. Irritable bowel syndrome can cause a variety of symptoms, from abdominal bloating and constipation to diarrhea. The symptoms may vary and may be related to other factors, such as stress or menstruation.

The first-line treatment of irritable bowel syndrome is increased consumption of dietary fiber to encourage normal bowel movements. Medications such as anti-spasmodics can be used to try to regulate bowel spasms. Laxatives may be used carefully if constipation is present.

Some drug treatments for an unstable bladder may worsen constipation (see p.45), and this must be kept in mind when treating irritable bowel syndrome.

BACK PROBLEMS

Lower back problems can cause pinching of the nerves supplying the bladder where they exit the spinal canal. This in turn can alter the function of these nerves and lead to difficulties in emptying the bladder. The first symptoms of a back problem may therefore appear to be caused by a urinary problem. Treatment of a bad back with properly supervised physical therapy can sometimes reduce the pressure caused by entrapment of the nerves and lead to the alleviation of symptoms.

FISTULAS

A fistula is an abnormal passage between two cavities, such as the bladder and the vagina, that can lead to incontinence. This passage can allow urine to leak directly into the vagina instead of being stored in the bladder.

Fistulas form for several reasons. In developed countries, the most common causes of fistulas are cancer and radiation therapy for cancer, because both weaken the muscles. Fistulas may also form after a surgical operation in which the surfaces have become damaged, particularly after a hysterectomy. In other parts of he world, the most common cause is an abnormally

The Effect of a Fistula

It is rare for a fistula, or abnormal connecting passage, to form between the bladder and the vagina. If it does, urine can pass directly into the vagina and leak out, causing incontinence.

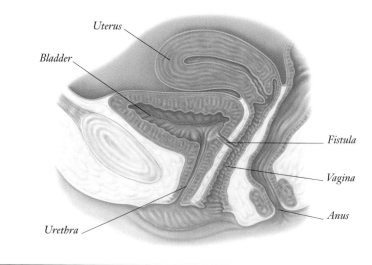

long labor leading to a pressure sore that erodes, forming a passage between the bladder and the vagina. Fistulas may also be congenital.

Fistulas are uncommon and require a specialist's care. In some cases they heal without an operation, but this process may take several weeks, during which a catheter is needed to keep the bladder empty. Operations for fistulas require great skill and postoperative care to help prevent recurrence.

CONGENITAL DEFECTS

Congenital defects are alterations in normal anatomy that are present at birth, such as an ectopic ureter. This is a condition in which the ureter (the tube that normally connects the bladder to the kidney) does not actually connect with the bladder. Instead, it connects directly to the vagina, which causes leaking because the bladder is bypassed. This is usually diagnosed and treated early in life.

KEY POINTS

- Other health problems may be associated with incontinence.
- Surgery should attempt to treat all problems at once.
- Treatment must be tailored to the individual's needs.

Managing the problem: aids and appliances

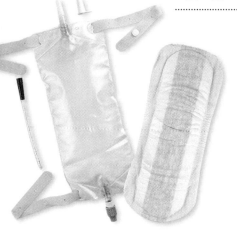

Over the past 20 years, there has been an increase in the number of companies producing incontinence products. The market for aids and appliances exists because most women prefer to deal with incontinence themselves rather than seek professional help.

INCONTINENCE AIDS
A variety of incontinence aids are available, including diapers and catheters.

Unfortunately, purchasing appliances for urinary incontinence without medical advice may prove expensive and ineffective if they are unsuitable for your condition or are not the correct size. Your doctor or one of the organizations dealing with incontinence (see Useful addresses, p.79) may be able to make recommendations about the purchase of these appliances to make your choice easier.

These products are designed to contain the problem sufficiently to allow "social" continence. There are many available, from panty liners allowing simple, discreet protection to fail-safe absorbent pads similar

What Do You Require?

There are many different products available to help you with your incontinence. The choice depends on these factors:

- What trouble does your incontinence cause?
- Do you leak small amounts often or large amounts infrequently?
- When does it trouble you? At night or only during exercise?
- How easy is it for you to change when you have leaked? Is it needed as a stopgap until you reach the toilet, or is it required to protect you for several hours?
- Do you need help to change or are you able to manage on your own?
- Can you easily remove a pad from a pouch within pants or are diapers easier?
- How important is it to have a discreet small pad that allows tight-fitting clothes?
- Do your size and shape make different products more acceptable or more difficult for you to use?

to diapers, and from underpads for seats and beds to catheters that keep the bladder permanently empty.

Most pharmacies stock a wide selection of products. The key to success in the choice of product lies in the assessment of your requirements. Your doctor or an incontinence organization is best equipped to provide advice regarding what can be done to limit the impact of incontinence on your lifestyle and to help you select the product best suited to your needs.

PANTY LINERS AND PADS

Panty liners offer the simplest means of protection. They are available at pharmacies and supermarkets, are unobtrusive, and are comfortable and easy to change. However, since they do not absorb urine very well, they may require frequent changing. The plastic backing may increase perspiration, which can be mistaken for leakage. They are an attractive option, however, because women often wear them under "normal" circumstances not necessarily associated with incontinence.

Pads that have a waterproof backing provide the wearer with greater security. They are more absorbent than panty liners but they may still allow leakage of urine around the edge. They also tend to be thicker, longer, and wider than panty liners. Some pads are shaped to allow a better fit.

Heavier pads are available for severe leakage problems; however for best results, stretch pants are required to hold them in position.

Considerations in Choice of Incontinence Aids

- Size
- Shape
- Reliability
- Quantity of urine held
- Odor
- Unobtrusiveness
- Comfort
- Skin irritability
- Price
- Accessibility and supply
- Disposable or reusable
- Ease of use and changing

MARSUPIAL PANTS

Marsupial pants are waterproof pants that contain a separate changeable pad within a pocket. This allows the pad to be changed independently of the pants. Urine drains through the porous layer of the pants into the pad. The major advantage of this system is that the pad does not have to be repositioned. This is useful for someone with impaired dexterity, who may find it difficult to reposition a pad after going to the bathroom. The drawback is that the inner lining is not changed after leakage, leaving a continuously wet layer next to the skin.

An increasing number of clothing companies are marketing underwear with either waterproof gussets or built-in pads. They are helpful in improving body image and allow women a wider choice of underwear.

DIAPERS

The most reliable of all systems is an all-in-one pad – disposable pants with a built-in pad. Improvements in the design have resulted in a much better fit and greater comfort. They are considerably lighter and better at containing leakage than the earlier versions.

MATTRESS COVERS

A wide variety of covers are available. The choice is dependent on the amount and frequency of leakage. A child who occasionally wets the bed will require a much lighter sheet than someone who continually empties his or her bladder. Newer designs of breathable fabrics tend to be more comfortable but also more expensive.

PROTECTING A BED
Place a protective covering on your child's bed if he or she is prone to bed-wetting.

UNDERPADS

There is a great variety of underpads available that can be used to protect furniture as well as beds. Underpads, composed of layers of absorbent material backed by a waterproof sheet, work by collecting leakage in a storage layer away from the skin. This protects the skin from sores caused by the irritation of long-term contact with urine.

KEY POINTS

- A wide range of products to help manage incontinence are available.
- Advice on products is available from the organizations listed in Useful addresses (p.79).
- The key to choosing the best product is accurate assessment of your requirements.

Glossary

Cystitis: Inflammation of the bladder. People frequently use the term to refer to a urinary tract infection accompanied by frequency, urgency, and dysuria.

Detrusor instability: An unstable bladder.

Detrusor muscle: The muscle in the bladder wall that contracts during urination.

Dysuria: Abnormal voiding that may be painful or difficult. This term is commonly used for pain during urination.

Enuresis: Bed-wetting, normally known as nocturnal enuresis because it occurs at night.

Frequency: Having to urinate more frequently than normal (normal is up to seven times a day or not more often than every two hours).

Hesitancy: A period of delay, with the sensation of having to void before urination begins.

Micturition: See voiding.

Nocturia: Having to get up more than once at night to urinate, usually affecting older individuals.

Perineum: The area between the vagina and the anus.

Prolapse: The displacement of a part of the body from its normal position. The term is usually used in association with changes of the pelvic organs "prolapsing" into the vagina.

Strangury: Gradual voiding accompanied by pain.

Stress incontinence: The leakage of urine caused by increased abdominal pressure (leakage with coughing, sneezing, or exercise).

Ultrasonography: A test using high-frequency sound waves to visualize deep structures of the body.

Ureter: The tube connecting the kidney to the bladder.

Urethra: The tube connecting the bladder to the outside.

Urethral sphincter: The bladder neck; the ring of muscles at the bottom of the bladder that opens during urination.

Urge incontinence: Urgency associated with leakage.

Urgency: The sudden and uncontrollable need to urinate.

Urine: Waste product of the body filtered by the kidneys.

Voiding: Emptying the bladder, also known as urination, micturition.

Useful addresses

American Association of Kidney Patients

Online: www.aakp.org

100 South Ashley Drive

Tampa, FL 33602

Tel: (800) 749-2257

E-mail: AAKPnat@aol.com

American Foundation for Urologic Disease

Online: www.afud.org

1126 North Charles Street

Baltimore, MD 21201

Tel: (410) 468-1800

E-mail: admin@afud.org

Home Delivery Incontinent Supplies

Online: www.nafc.org

1215 Dillman Industrial Court

Olivette, MO 63132

Tel: (800) 2MY-HOME (269-4663)

Interstitial Cystitis Association (ICA)

Online: www.ichelp.org

51 Monroe Street

Rockville, MD 20850

Tel: (301) 610-5300

Fax: (301) 610-5308

E-mail: icmail@ichelp.org

National Association for Continence

Online: www.nafc.org

PO Box 8310

Spartanburg, SC 29305

Tel: (800) BLADDER

Tel: (864) 579-7900

Fax: (864) 579-7902

National Kidney Foundation Information Center

Online: www.kidney.org

30 East 33rd Street

New York, NY 10016

Tel: (800) 488-2277

National Kidney and Urologic Diseases Information Clearinghouse

Online: www.niddk.nih.gov/health/kidney/nkudic.htm

3 Information Way

Bethesda, MD 20892-3560

Tel: (800) 654-4415

E-mail: nkudic@info.niddk.nih.gov

Simon Foundation for Continence

PO Box 835

Wilmette, IL 60091

Tel: (800) 23-SIMON

Notes

Notes

Notes

Notes

Notes

Index

Acknowledgments

PUBLISHER'S ACKNOWLEDGMENTS
Dorling Kindersley Publishing, Inc. would like to thank the following for their help and participation in this project:

Managing Editor Stephanie Jackson; **Managing Art Editor** Nigel Duffield; **Editorial Assistance** Mary Lindsay, Irene Pavitt; Design Revolution; **Design Assistance** Sarah Hall, Marianne Markham, Design Revolution, Chris Walker; **Production** Michelle Thomas, Elizabeth Cherry.

Consultancy Dr. Tony Smith, Dr. Sue Davidson; **Indexing** Indexing Specialists, Hove; **Administration** Christopher Gordon.

Illustrations (p.28, p.30, p.33, p.34, p.38, p.41, p.57, p.67, p.70) ©Philip Wilson.

Picture Research Angela Anderson, Andy Sansom; **Picture Librarian** Charlotte Oster.

PICTURE CREDITS
The publisher would like to thank the following for their kind permission to reproduce their photographs. Every effort has been made to trace the copyright holders. Dorling Kindersley apologizes for any unintentional omissions and would be pleased, in any such cases, to add an acknowledgment in future editions.

APM Studios p.40; **Art Directors Photo Library** p.52; **Science Photo Library** p.12 (CNRI); **Telegraph Colour Library** p.80.

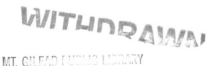